Copyright © 2012, All Rights Reserved

All rights reserved. No part of this e-book may be reproduced or transmitted in any form or by any means, electronic or mechanical, including photocopying, recording, or by any information storage and retrieval system, without the expressed written permission from Jonathan Haas.

Disclaimer:

You must get your physician's approval before beginning this exercise program. These recommendations are not medical guidelines but are for educational purposes only.

You must consult your physician prior to starting this program or if you have any medical condition or injury that contraindicates physical activity. This program is designed for healthy individuals 18 years and older only.
The information in this e manual is meant to supplement, not replace, proper exercise training. All forms of exercise pose some inherent risks. The author advises readers to take full responsibility for their safety and know their limits. Before practicing the exercises in this e manual, be sure that your equipment is well maintained, and do not take risks beyond your level of experience, aptitude, training and fitness. The exercises in this book are not in-tended as a substitute for any exercise routine or treatment that may have been prescribed by your physician.

See your physician before starting any exercise or nutrition program. If you are taking any medications, you must talk to your physician before starting any exercise program,
If you experience any light headedness, dizziness, or shortness of breath while exercising, stop the movement and consult a physician.

This program is dedicated to my Dad, Peter Haas, Jr.

True strength is measured by more than an ability to move heavy weight.

Happy Father's Day, June 2012.

"Promise Yourself"

To be so strong that nothing
can disturb your peace of mind.
To talk health, happiness, and prosperity
to every person you meet.

To make all your friends feel
that there is something in them
To look at the sunny side of everything
and make your optimism come true.

To think only the best, to work only for the best,
and to expect only the best.
To be just as enthusiastic about the success of others
as you are about your own.

To forget the mistakes of the past
and press on to the greater achievements of the future.
To wear a cheerful countenance at all times
and give every living creature you meet a smile.

To give so much time to the improvement of yourself
that you have no time to criticize others.
To be too large for worry, too noble for anger, too strong for fear,
and too happy to permit the presence of trouble.

To think well of yourself and to proclaim this fact to the world,
not in loud words but great deeds.
To live in faith that the whole world is on your side
so long as you are true to the best that is in you.

— Christian D. Larson

> *"Dad Strength, when being strong for others isn't just a one-time thing, but a lifetime commitment."*
> - *Jon Haas*

Welcome to Dad Strength!

My own personal quest for **Dad Strength** began years ago when my eldest daughter, Caitlin, at 3 years old asked me, "Dad, will you always be able to pick me up and carry me?"

My immediate response to her was, "Of course, baby. Daddy will always be able to carry you."

But the little one persisted, "Even when I'm older and bigger? Even when you're old and I'm 100?"

To which I replied, "Always. No matter how big you get or how old I get, I will always be strong enough to carry you."

And I was serious. What began as a promise to a wide-eyed 3 year old who probably never actually expected me to be able to keep it, has become a lifelong quest for **Dad Strength**.

Prior to getting married and having children, my pursuit of strength, health, fitness, and even martial art was always for myself. Nothing really wrong with that, per se - it was a source of pride to be a strong, fit warrior, but it was only about me. Now, as a man with a wife and 2 beautiful girls, I find my pursuit of those things stronger than ever, but the emphasis behind why I do it has changed. Now I train to be strong for them. I have found that being strong for others is an incredibly powerful motivating factor, much greater than just for me.

What's Wrong with Men Today?

There's no denying it, men as a whole are getting weaker. And to our own detriment as a society, as a nation, and as a world, we are progressively getting more and more comfortable with our weakness. It has become habitual for us to, and what is habitual becomes normal. But to be weak is not normal and should not be accepted as such. The sad fact though is that it's considered abnormal to see a man in good physical condition over 40. Sometimes even over 30. When did this happen? Why did we as a society allow this to happen? But even more importantly, what are we going to do about it?

As a Dad you must be strong for others. Your hands have to channel strength to support, to help, to pick up, to carry and share burdens. From strength comes confidence. Brilliant self-confidence inspires others. Confidence radiates out like a beacon which draws others to you and which others draw support from.

Why Dad Strength?

Remember back when you were a little kid and your father always looked like this physically imposing, towering figure of a man? You had this perception of your dad as a super-human figure who could pick you up over his head and put you on his strong shoulders to be able to see the world. Standing on the shoulders of giants, indeed.

How about when you and a friend would get into a little scuffle at the playground and one of you, almost without fail, would whip out the classic taunt – "well, my Dad can beat up your Dad!" The both of you had this firm, unshakable faith in each of your fathers' ability to protect, defend, and keep you safe from any and all harm, including fighting other kid's dads for dominion over the playground.

This image of your dad's strength and physical potency continued unabated for most of your childhood, right?

But then what happened? We grew up. Got taller. Got stronger. Matured. And gradually began to see that Dad, while still the man you learn from, look up to, and turn to for help in times of need, is just a normal human being (albeit, an exceptional one at that – hi Dad!).

What if, as *your* children grow, mature, and get stronger, moving from children to teens to adults, their perception of *your* Dad Strength never faded? What if their amazement at *your* physical capabilities never waned? What if *you* were able to not only maintain (since we are either moving forwards or backwards, but are never really static) but increase strength, power, and ability, as *you* age? What if *you* could be not only fitter, stronger, and healthier, but better?

This **Dad Strength program** will take a holistic approach to developing sustainable fitness. You will learn how to:

- Stand tall
- Move with power, coordination, and grace.
- Not allow middle age to expand your middle.
- Attack weakness and lack of energy.
- Reduce or alleviate low back pain.
- Reduce strain and increase healthy stress.

- Move with dignity and purpose
- You will learn how to get strong. Stay strong.

~ You will not go gently into that good night! ~

Start with Sustainable Fitness

In recent years super-intense workout programs seem to be all the rage. The crazier, more insane it is, the more people flock to it. But are these programs sustainable for the long haul? Intensity must be balance with recovery to allow for adaptation and growth to occur. No gains happen during the workout itself. All of the benefits derived from the work happened during the recovery period. It can also be argued that recovery aids in allowing the body to perform at greater and greater levels of intensity.

This program incorporates daily joint mobility work as a form of pre-habilitation, or injury prevention. It then further balances effort with recovery to guarantee continuous upward progress without being sidelined by pain and injury. You will work hard here, but rest hard as well!

"Do not pray for easy lives. Pray to be stronger men"

- **John F. Kennedy**

Phase I – Reclaim Your Body

Phase I will be about relearning how to live as a physical being. You will move, stand, stretch, and breath perhaps like you've never done before. You will feel healthier, more alert, and more alive. And this is just the start.

For the first week of this program just perform the mobility exercises, yoga postures, and breathing exercises on a daily basis to begin to reclaim your health, strength, and energy. The entire thing will only take about 20 minutes.

Mobility is where it all happens. We must unload areas of chronic tightness and tension before adding the stress of exercises otherwise all we are doing is reinforcing those pre-existing patterns of tension. Mobility training will move your joints through their natural range of motion to open up the joints and recover your full range of motion (ROM).

Remember, if you don't move it you lose it!

Benefits of Mobility Training

Let's list out some of the benefits of mobility training:

- Lubricates joints and allows them to receive nutrition through synovial fluid
- Aids in removal of toxins
- Reduces joint pain and inflammation
- Increases range of motion (flexibility in motion)
- Increases energy by reducing unconsciously held tension
- Prehab for injury prevention
- Mobility is foundation of all sport, athletic, and martial movement
- Decreased mobility leads to increased pain and stiffness

In order to get the most bang for our buck we will concentrate on the main problem areas: neck, shoulders, back, chest, hips/pelvis, and knees – move it or lose it

Recovering Mobility

On a daily basis, perform the following exercises for 10 to 12 reps each. For greater results do them multiple times a day. They will only take a few minutes to perform, but the returns will be huge.

Neck:

1. Up/Down – lift up from crown of head; slide down along plane of jaw.
2. Left/Right – turn head as far left as possible without pain, turn as far right as possible.
3. Full circles in both directions.

Shoulders:

1. Roll both shoulders – lift shoulders up towards ears, roll backward fully articulating the range of motion (ROM), drop them down as far as comfortable, then repeat by rolling forward.
2. Alternate shoulder rolls – roll left shoulder back as described above while pushing right shoulder forward then switch.
3. Swing both arms as fast as possible wind milling them forward then backward.

Chest:

1. Inhale as you lift the chest up at a 45 degree angle
2. Exhale and stretch arms straight out in front as you move backwards reaching with mid-back.

Hips/Pelvis:

1. Circle hips clockwise and counter-clockwise.
2. Tilt pelvis forward and backward

3. Tilt pelvis left to right.

Knees:

1. Put feet together, bend knees and place hands on knee caps.
2. Rotate knees circularly in both directions.

Spine:

1. Keep the spine straight and fold forward at the hips
2. Rotate around to the left and back to center, then forward and around to the right.
3. Keep the spine straight and fold backward at the hips, then rotate around to the left and back to center, then forward and around to the right.

Stand Like a Man

Presence begins with posture. You cannot have a commanding presence with stooped shoulders, rounded back, and sunken chest. Your posture should exude confidence and strength. The way you stand should cause other people to look at you with respect before you even speak. Allow your posture to create an impression.

In order to this you must learn how to stack the bones to be anti-gravity. No leaning. No canting the hip to one side or the other. Your body will rest on its own structure.

The cadence for how you will stand is:

- Crown up
- Chin down
- Shoulders down and back
- Elbows down
- Spine straight – no pelvis tuck or arch
- Knees slightly bent – never locked
- Mid-foot balance

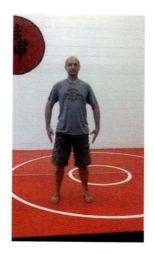

Stand proud and strong, Dad!

Yoga for Dad

Here we will utilize basic yoga postures with a focus on increasing flexibility and strength, opening up the chest, breathing deeply, and beginning to bring balance back to the body.

Every activity that we repeat consistently causes an adaptation in the body. The critical thing to note here is that it does not matter at all how we value this adaptation. It can be something that we want like how healthy exercise increases lean muscle mass and burns excess fat, or it can be something we do not want like how eating junk food to an extreme causes our body to adapt by putting on weight. Both of these are examples of activities that cause adaptations in the body. Sitting for extended periods of time whether behind a desk or on a couch also causes specific adaptations in the body. We tend to become chair shaped or couch shaped; our bodies adopt a rounded back, slumped shoulders posture while standing and performing activities other than sitting. In order to bring our bodies back to balance, we must compensate specifically for the typical posture held when sitting.

Yoga is designed to bring your body back to balance. Don't worry, I'm not about to ask you to jump into a Power Yoga class for Dad's. Not unless you want to, anyway. What I am going to have you do is take about 10 minutes during the day and use just a few simple yoga postures to help bring your body back to equilibrium. These postures will help to prevent, or relieve, the back and neck pain that tend to be associated with long term sitting, whether due to working on a computer, sitting on the couch in front of the TV. An added benefit is that we will also open up your chest and lungs to improve your breathing pattern and help reduce stress.

On a daily basis, perform each of the below yoga postures for 30 to 60 seconds each. Emphasis on deep breathing in through the nose and out through the mouth. The sequence may be done multiple times a day for greater benefit.

Upward Facing Dog

In this posture only the hands and tops of feet are touching the mat. Lift up from crown of head, push down into mat. Tighten glutes to protect low back. Inhale deeply through nose, exhale through the mouth.

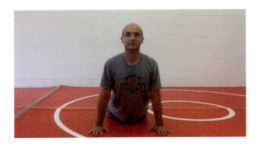 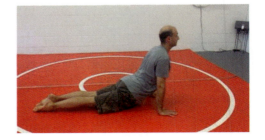

Downward Facing Dog

From the previous Upward Facing Dog posture, push back rolling over tops of feet. Straighten knees, tighten quads, and tilt pelvis towards the ceiling. Core is tight. Inhale deeply through nose, exhale through the mouth.

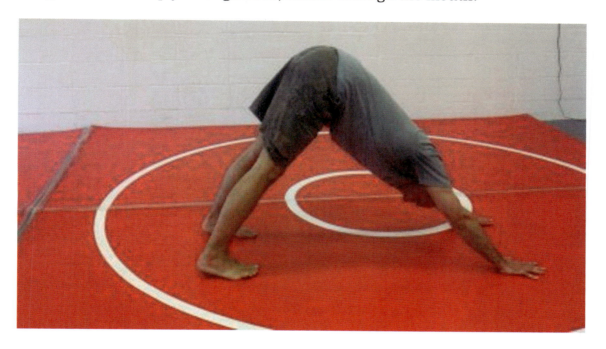

Shoulder Bridge

Lie on your back; bring feet as close to butt as possible while staying flat on mat. Exhale and drive hips up. Tighten glutes, tighten core. Inhale deeply through nose, exhale through the mouth.

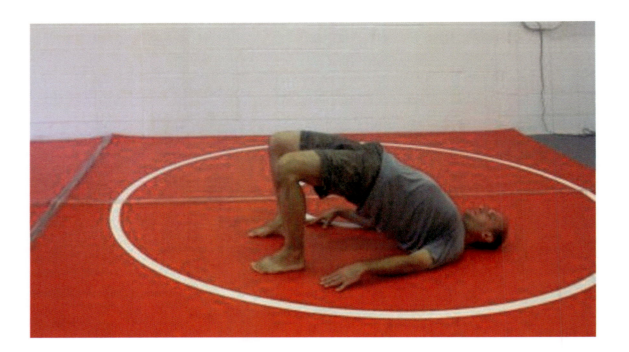

Wind Removing Pose

From the previous Shoulder Bridge posture, lower hips and hug knees tightly into chest. Press low back into mat to flatten it.

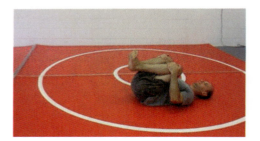

Sleeping Warrior

From a kneeling posture, fold forward at the hips; straighten arms and try to pull mat towards you. This is a great stretch for the shoulders and upper back. Inhale deeply through nose, exhale through the mouth.

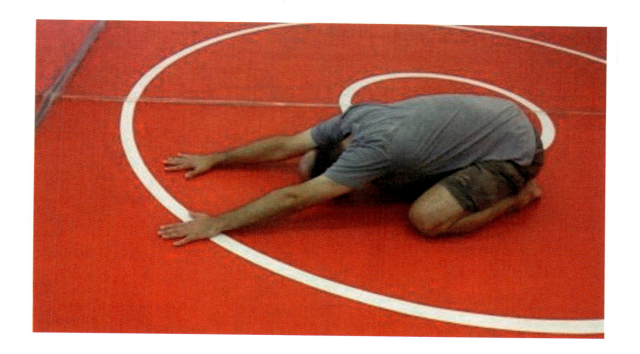

Seated Spinal Twist

Sit up with legs straight out in front of you. Cross one leg over and hug knee tightly to your chest. Twist at the waist towards the planted foot. Inhale deeply through nose, exhale through the mouth.

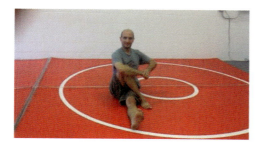 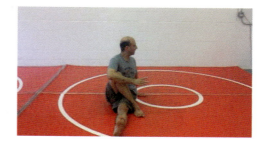

Right and Left Leg Forward Lunges

Start with a right leg forward lunge. Contract the left glute, lift tall from the crown of head, exhale and lean forward. Inhale deeply through nose, exhale through the mouth. Switch to left lead lunge.

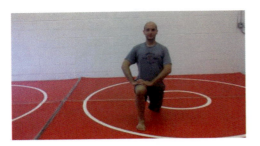

Left and Right Side Bends

Stand up with feet together and knees locked. Tighten quads, core, and glutes. Inhale hands up above your head. Exhale and lean to one side. Inhale hands back up and then go to other side on an exhale.

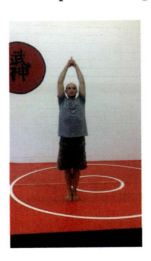 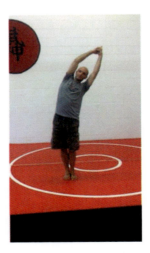

Dad's Breath

Most men don't pay too much attention to breathing. It goes on all day, every day pretty much without thought. It is basically like a process on a computer running in the background. Maybe the only time it's noticed is when there's an issue. But, we are going to bring that process to the forefront and start paying attention to it.

You may not be aware that breathing is a bridge between our voluntary and autonomic nervous systems. Meaning breath is plugged into both. The autonomic system will keep you breathing continuously without your conscious control, or sometimes, without even your awareness of it going on. But, you also have the power to override that control and decide at any moment to take a deep breath or hold your breath. What does this mean to you though, right? Well, here's what it means, you have the power, at any time, to consciously choose to influence things like your heart rate and blood pressure which are not under your conscious control. Now that's fascinating to me! Because breath is tied into both systems it can be used like a bridge to gain access to aspects of your body that you cannot directly control. How do we do this?

Try This Experiment

Take your pulse. Count beats for 10 seconds then multiply by 6. If you're sitting and relaxed, that number should be your resting heart rate. Now, inhale as deeply as possible and hold your breath and tense your whole body for a few seconds. Are you red in the face? Take your pulse again. What happened? Your heart rate jumped up and your blood pressure spiked right along with it, right?

Now try exhaling for a count of 6, but don't inhale yet. Extend the pause before the inhale a little bit. Feel more relaxed? Check your pulse. It should have dropped. Pretty cool, eh? And this is just the beginning.

Relaxing Breath (Square Breathing)

This is very similar to the experiment we did above. The basic premise of our ability to influence the autonomic nervous system is that inhalation increases heart rate, which subsequently increase blood pressure, to a slight degree, while exhalation lowers heart rate and blood pressure to a slight degree. During our normal cycle of breathing, these changes are too minute to register, or even notice. But, by gradually lengthening our breath and extending the pause before inhaling and exhaling, we compound the effect.

1. Begin by exhaling through the mouth for 5 seconds.
2. Do not inhale. Try to extend the breath pause for 5 seconds.
3. Before tension begins to creep in, inhale for 5 seconds.
4. Hold the breath on the inhale for 5 seconds.
5. Repeat the cycle 10 times.
6. As this becomes easier, and your capacity expands, try increasing the duration to 6, 7, 8 seconds.

Restoring Breath

This one is literally a life saver when doing high intensity workouts! It can be used in between exercises as well as in between sets, during the rest period, and at the end of the workout to normalize breathing and dramatically lower heart rate.

1. Forcefully exhale as deeply as possible by rolling your shoulders forward, tilting the pelvis up, and contracting the core strongly. Attempt to pull the navel to the spine!
2. Pause before the inhale for a few seconds.
3. As stated above, do not actively inhale. Allow the breath to be sucked back in through the nose as your body returns to a natural standing posture.
4. Repeat for about 60 seconds, or as long as needed.

Dad's Quick Morning Recharge

This is a routine I have been using successfully for years to shake out the cobwebs and get me moving on the mornings when just a cup of coffee isn't going to do it. It's not your fault, and bear in mind – some people just aren't morning people.

Back when I was travelling for weeks on end and putting in long hours every day for consulting work this routine was my morning staple in the hotel room before meeting my colleagues for breakfast. I find it most effective on the mornings when I am most tired. Just as an aside, it doesn't have to be used only in the mornings; it has benefits any time of the day when you need a little pick me up. One caution, and although this should be obvious I'll say it anyway, don't do it before going to bed – you won't sleep!

Energizing Breath

In this breathing exercise we will utilize a protocol founded by yoga and improved upon by Russian sport science and martial art. Here the breath is divided into 3 levels: clavicular (upper level), intercostal (mid-level), and diaphragmatic (lower level). This exercise will focus only on the clavicular, or upper level.

1. Exhale through the mouth in a short, quick burst by compressing the upper chest.
2. Do not actively inhale. Allow the inhale to happen by relaxing the muscles in the chest.
3. Repeat rapidly 20 to 40 times.
4. Build up to where you can perform continuously for 60 seconds.
5. If you become dizzy, stop and sit down!

Slap Yourself Silly!

This is actually an ancient Qigong exercise designed to improve circulation and disperse stagnant energy. The execution is pretty simple. You may want to avoid practicing this in public though!

1. Gently, but vigorously, slap your shoulders, upper back, and lower back with the palms of the hands.
2. Then slap down the inside of one arm and up the outside. Switch arms.
3. Slap down the outside of both legs – you can slap a little harder here – and up the inside.

Enjoy and Wake Up!

Phase II – Building Dad Strength

In Phase II we will begin the process of building whole body strength. In order for the body to work as an integrated whole, it must be trained together. Since the combined power of the whole body is much greater than the sum of its individual parts, there will be no isolation of parts or muscle groups.

The synergistic effect of the mobility plus the yoga plus the strength training will have a system-wide impact on your body. Not only will you experience and increase in strength, but also in coordination, flexibility, posture, endurance, and overall ease of movement.

This type of training will help alleviate pain and allow you to gradually restore and then refine your natural strength, grace, and carriage.

Weeks 2 to 4

Workout Notes:

Perform workouts on non-consecutive days. Continue to do joint mobility on a daily basis, preferably in the AM as part of your Morning Recharge Routine.

Sub Max (SM) effort means do not go all out; leave 1 to 2 reps in the tank.

Max Effort (ME) means do as many reps as possible in that set.

Supersets are alternating between 2 or more exercises for the duration of the set. The exercises will often be placed as antagonistic movements opposite each other, like a push-pull combination.

For all squats keep weight on heels, squat with butt back and knees out.

Always exhale on effort and focus on keeping the core braced tightly on every exercise.

Workout # 1

Warm-up

Use joint mobility routine and energizing breath described above as a warm-up for all workouts.

The Main Workout

1) Bodyweight Squats 4 x 15 (60 second rest)
2) Pushups 4 x SM (60 second rest)
3) Straight Leg Sit-ups 3 x 10 (60 second rest)
4) Recline Row 3 x SM (60 second rest)
5) Alternating Forward Lunges 3 x 15/15 60 second rest)

Straight Leg Sit-ups – Lie on your back, exhale and contract the core, begin to sit up slowly keeping your spine straight. Inhale at the top of the movement. Exhale again and slowly lie back down.

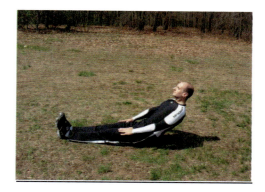

Recline Row – This can be easily replicated by attaching a rope to a portable pull-up bar or tree branch. Portable pull-up bars are found in almost any sporting goods store or on Amazon.

Dumbbell rows may be substituted for recline rows should no rope or pull-up bar be available.

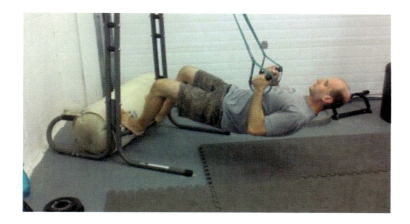

Cool Down

Use this cool down routine for all workouts.

(The Restoring Breath can be used in between exercises as well as in between sets, during the rest period, and at the end of the workout to normalize breathing and dramatically lower heart rate.)

Upward Facing Dog – hold for 30 seconds
Downward Facing Dog – hold for 30 seconds
Sleeping Warrior – hold for 30 seconds
Shoulder Bridge – hold for 30 seconds
Right leg forward Lunge – hold for 15 seconds
Left leg forward Lunge – hold for 15 seconds
Standing Side Bend – hold for 15 seconds left/right

Repeat 1 – 3 times, as needed.

Workout #2

The Main Workout

1) Walking Forward Lunges 4 x 15/15 (60 second rest)
2) Pull-up 3 x SM first set: palm out, second set: palm in, third set: one out, one in (60 second rest)
3) V-Ups 3 x 10 (60 second rest)
4) Close Grip Push-ups (fingers touching in a diamond shape) 3 x SM

V-ups - Lie flat on your back with arms stretched out above your head. Exhale, contract your core, and lift both arms and legs together to form your body into a "V" shape. Inhale as you lie back down and repeat. Make sure to control this movement with appropriate core tension to avoid "flopping" back onto the ground.

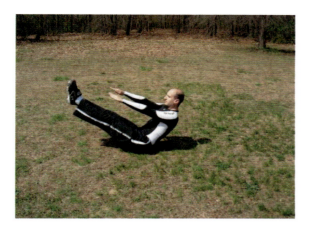

Workout #3

The Main Workout

1) Bodyweight Squats 4 x 15
2A) Mixed Grip Push-ups 4 x SM (change hand position each set)
2B) Recline Rows 4 x SM

Finisher – Plank hold for time

Weeks 5 to 7

Workout Notes:

Perform workouts on non-consecutive days. Continue to do joint mobility on a daily basis, preferably in the AM as part of your Morning Recharge Routine.

Sub Max (SM) effort means do not go all out; leave 1 to 2 reps in the tank.

Max Effort (ME) means do as many reps as possible in that set.

Supersets are alternating between 2 or more exercises for the duration of the set. The exercises will often be placed as antagonistic movements opposite each other, like a push-pull combination.

For all squats keep weight on heels, squat with butt back and knees out.

Always exhale on effort and focus on keeping the core braced tightly on every exercise.

Workout #1

<u>The Main Workout</u>

1A) Bodyweight Squats 4 x 15
1B) Push-ups 4 x SM
(Rest 60 seconds)
2A) Alternating Forward Lunges 3 x 15
2B) Dips on chair or bed 3 x 10-15
(Rest 60 seconds)
3) Core work 3 x 10-15 (first set: V-ups, second set: Knee Tucks, third set: Supermans)

Knee Tucks - Begin seated with legs pulled into chest. Extend legs straight out in front without your feet touching the ground. Exhale, contract your core, and pull your legs back into your chest.

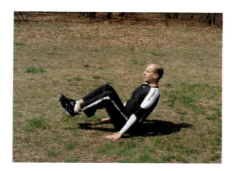

Supermans – Lie on your stomach with arms straight out in front of you. Exhale, contract the core and raise both arms and both legs at the same time

Workout #2

<u>The Main Workout</u>

1A) Super Slow Push-ups (15 seconds down/15 seconds up) 4 x 5
1B) Super Slow Squats (15 seconds down/15 seconds up) 4 x 5
1C) Super Slow Leg Raises (15 seconds down/15 seconds up) 4 x 5
(Rest 2 – 3 minutes)
2) Push-ups 1 x ME
(Rest 1 minute)
3) Bodyweight Squats 1 x ME
(Rest 1 Minute)
4) Leg Raises 1 x ME

Workout #3

The Main Workout

1) Bodyweight Squats 20, 15, 10, 5 (60 second rest)
2) Push-ups 10, 8, 6, 4 (60 second rest)
3) Reverse Lunges 4 x 15 (60 second rest)
4) Plank 3 x 30 second holds

"Pain is temporary. It may last a minute, or an hour, or a day, or a year, but eventually it will subside and something else will take its place. If I quit, however, it lasts forever."

Lance Armstrong

Phase III - From Dad to Super Dad

Phase III will combine both strength & conditioning for greater gains. The conditioning aspect of our program for this phase will utilize High Intensity Interval Training (HIIT). HIIT is perhaps one of the best ways to train for fat loss and overall endurance. It will enhance all 3 energy systems in the body (2 anaerobic and 1 aerobic), as well as prime the nervous system to recover automatically during lulls in activity. Simply put, HIIT alternates periods of high intensity exercise with periods of rest and recovery. It can be performed with almost any exercise and can be utilized both with and without equipment. The variety and adaptability of this style of training is second to none in results.

The Body's 3 Energy Systems

To briefly summarize, the body has three energy systems, 2 anaerobic, or non-oxidative, and 1 aerobic, that serve to create ATP (adenosine triphosphate). ATP is utilized by every cell in your body; it fuels muscular contractions, cognitive processes, and internal regulatory functions. Both anaerobic systems fuel maximally intensive activity, while the aerobic system fuels sustained low to moderate level activity.

The ATP-PC system provides immediately available energy for high intensity efforts from ATP stored within the muscles. This system is the most powerful, but least enduring of the three, lasting only about 10 to 30 seconds max.

The Glycolytic system, the second most powerful, is only slightly more enduring than the ATP-PC system. It derives energy from glycogen stored in the muscles and liver converting it to ATP in a process called glycolysis. Its capacity is approximately 90 to 120 seconds. Rest intervals allow the body to recuperate and restore ATP.

Lastly, the Aerobic system uses proteins, fats, and carbohydrates to produce ATP. As the intensity of the effort increases, the aerobic system relies more on glycogen for energy. If the intensity continues to increase, the anaerobic systems must kick-in to provide energy. The important idea to realize here is that all 3 energy systems are always supplying the body with the energy it needs for any activity, at any level of intensity. It's just that one may be more dominant than the other 2 at a specific time.

Tabata Protocol

No discussion of interval training would be complete without touching on the Tabata Protocol. Dr. Izumi Tabata at the National Institute of Fitness and Sports in Tokyo, Japan performed perhaps the most well-known study on interval training. A group exercising with moderate intensity endurance training was compared to another group using high intensity intermittent training. Each group exercised 5 days a week. The moderate intensity group exercised for 60 minutes, at 70% VO2 max. The high intensity group did 8 intervals of 20 seconds, followed by 10 seconds of recovery. They operated at 170% VO2 max.

After 6 weeks, both groups experienced improvements in maximal oxygen uptake. The biggest difference between them was that only the high intensity group gained improvement in anaerobic capacity. The high intensity group actually realized a 28% increase in anaerobic capacity AND a 14% increase in VO2max. So, the study concluded that high intensity intermittent training can improve both the anaerobic and aerobic systems simultaneously.

Weeks 8 to 10 (and Beyond!)

Workout #1 – Strength Focus

Repeat workout #1 from weeks 2 to 4 above as the strength workout. Gauge your progress!

1) Bodyweight Squats 4 x 15 (60 second rest)
2) Pushups 4 x SM (60 second rest)
3) Straight Leg Sit-ups 3 x 10 (60 second rest)
4) Recline Row 3 x SM (60 second rest)
5) Alternating Forward Lunges 3 x 15/15 60 second rest)

Workout #2 – Conditioning Focus

Perform each exercise for 30 seconds. No rest between exercises. Complete 3 to 5 rounds, rest 60 seconds between rounds.

1) Jumping Jacks
2) Burpees

3) Running in place

4) Push-ups

5) Bodyweight Squats

6) Mountain Climbers

"He who has a why to live for can bear almost any how."
-Friedrich Nietzsche

Workout #3 – Conditioning Focus

Perform each exercise using Tabata protocol (8 x 20 secs/ 10 secs)

1) Alternating Lunges (60 second rest)

2) Push-ups (60 second rest)

3) Lateral Jumps (60 second rest)

4) Burpees (60 second rest)

Finish with core work 3 x 10-15 (first set: V-ups, second set: Knee Tucks, third set: Supermans)

A Quick Word on Nutrition

Rather than an extensive dissertation on nutrition, I will sum up my dietary advice in a single phrase:

Eat Like a Caveman Dad!

You see, prior to the Agricultural Revolution some 10,000 years ago (give or take), all humans – everyone on the planet – ate basically the same diet. Of course there were some variations due to geography, climate, and seasons, yes, but basically the same diet. And what if I told you that this one diet kept our caveman (and woman) ancestors leaner, stronger, fitter, and even healthier than we are today? It enabled them to survive and thrive for over 2 million years.

Our genes have remained virtually unchanged since pre-agricultural times. We are quite literally cavemen in business suits – some of us more so than others! The premise of the Cave-Dad Diet is that our current genetic expression is influenced, positively or negatively, by our lifestyle. So that how we eat, how we exercise (or don't), how we rest, play, and sleep all combine to create the body we have today. This means that we literally have the ability to optimize our genetic potential one forkful at a time. .

Grains and other processed foods at the top of the list of things to avoid. Yes, even the supposedly healthy, whole grains. Why? Simply because humans did not evolve to digest grains properly. They make us fat and unhealthy. Remember our genes have not changed since pre-Agricultural times.

There are many benefits to eating this way, including a naturally lean body, acne-free skin, improved athletic performance and recovery, and relief from numerous metabolic-related and autoimmune diseases.

Cave-Dad Diet Summary

- You can eat all lean meat, fish, seafood & eggs
- You can eat all non-starchy seasonal vegetables
- Plenty of seasonal fruit
- Moderate healthy fats
- Moderate nuts and seeds
- No grains or cereals at all
- No legumes
- No processed foods
- No sugars.
- No artificial sweeteners. These are not food!

In answer to your question, yes, alcohol is allowed in moderation. But remember, if you want to get rid of that beer belly, you should probably limit your consumption of beer. Additionally, the hops in beer has been linked to increased estrogen levels, certainly not what we want!

Too Busy to Train?

These days everyone is short on time. Most are content to allow the daily grind and family time to fill their days while lamenting about the fact that they have no time for working out. The complaints are common and heard often. But somehow these same people are able to find time to watch an hour or more of TV every night before going to bed. Don't worry, I'm not going to ask you to forego your favorite Thursday night TV episode in favor of hitting the gym for an hour, I'm just using the ability to watch TV as an example of "finding time".

Here's a list of 8 ways for these busy people to fit in their fitness and reclaim a healthy lifestyle.

1. Plan it out. Scheduling is the key to successful time management. Look at your weekly calendar and plan to exercise just as you would plan an important client meeting, a lunch with an old friend, or coaching your kid's Little League team.

2. Exercise wherever you are. Joint mobility sessions can be done at your desk.

3. Work in an office building? Take the stairs instead of the elevator. See how fast you can make it to your floor – beat those lazy suckers in the elevator to your floor!

4. Have a lunch break? Go outside and go for a walk. 10 minutes in the fresh air will do wonders for you. Eat at your desk while you work and then go for a walk. Want to make your walk more productive? Try inhaling for 5 steps, holding your breath on the inhale for 5 steps, exhaling for 5 steps, then holding the breath after the exhale for 5 steps. When you can comfortably do that for the entire duration of your walk, increase to 6, 8, 10 steps!

5. Get up earlier and do it! ****warning – this one requires effort and commitment!!****

6. Spend quality time exercising and playing with your kids. Show them what **Dad Strength** can do!

7. Brief workouts. Got a spare 15 minutes? Bring the intensity and lose the long, boring workouts.

8. Isometrics. These require very little time to be effective, need no equipment, and can be done literally anywhere.

Awaken the Man

Comfortably slumbering under the influence of the drug that is modern society, the true power of man lies dormant. Too much of the wrong foods have made him sluggish and their excesses have made him round. Too much sitting, whether it be in an office laboring behind a keyboard, or on a couch relaxing from that labor in front of a television, has made him weak and brittle. Too much time indoors has taken the natural healthy glow and replaced it with a pasty, snow white tan gained under the glare of a fluorescent sun. Too many worries and stresses about how to have more, or keep it, have robbed him of his real sleep and etched artificial lines across his forehead and bags under his eyes. (Are we still worried about the zombie apocalypse? Hell, it may already be happening and we don't even know it!)

Yet with all this, the poor fool doesn't even know he's slumbering – he thinks he's awake! What's even more the tragedy is he thinks this is all there is.

Wake Up!

There's an alarm clock blaring somewhere in your head, sounding a clarion call. It's faint and far off, I know, but listen. Focus. Hear it. It gets louder. The call becomes clearer. Wake UP!

> *"You just don't understand*
> *this is how you're being defined*
> *it's time to awaken the man*
> *from the din within your mind"*
> *- Awaken the Man by Din Within*

It's a simple 3 step process:

1) Free your mind. Realize that there's much more than this.
2) Awaken your spirit. Have passion for something, anything!
3) Make fierce your body.

This physical body, our only real possession, is an amazing thing. Use it. Test it. Push the perceived barriers of it and then blow past them. It's a shame to waste it. Move. Lift something heavy. Sprint for all you're worth. Climb high. Throw far. Leap over something. Crawl under something. Fight. Train. Breath deeply. Live.

"It's time to Awaken The Man who hides behind the lies"

Open your eyes. Really see yourself. When you look in the mirror are you satisfied with who you are and what you've become? If not, why the hell not? Do something about it now. Live with commitment.

Wake UP!

Bonus Special Report:

10 Ways to Increase Testosterone Naturally!

Low testosterone has virtually become an epidemic today. Studies have shown that men, on average, have only about ½ the testosterone that they had 50 years ago. Think that your grandfather was stronger, tougher, and manlier than you? You're probably right, but here's how to fix it!

1. Get plenty of Omega-3 fatty acid. Take your fish oil.

2. Make sure to get at least 3,000 to 5,000 IU of Vitamin D3 per day.

3. Take a 10 minute cold shower (yes, cold!) 2 times a day – in the morning when you wake up and at night before bed.

4. Eat nuts – almonds and Brazil nuts are best.

5. No processed foods. These franken-foods are killing us.

6. Strength training and high intensity interval training (this program!)

7. Eat organic foods as much as possible.

8. Eat healthy fats – grass fed beef and coconut milk are great ones.

9. Keep your cell phone away from your "boys".

10. Have more sex!

About Jon

First and foremost, I am a husband and father of 2 beautiful girls!

Jon Haas is the founder of Warrior Fitness Training Systems. He is a certified Underground Strength Coach and has been involved in the martial arts for over 30 years.

Jon has been training in the Budō Taijutsu arts of the Bujinkan for more than 22 years and is currently ranked as a Kudan (9th degree black belt) under Jack Hoban Shidōshi. He is also the author of the book, *Warrior Fitness: Conditioning for Martial Arts*.

Jon is a certified conflict resolutions specialist through Resolution Group International (RGI).

Additional Recommended Resources

Warrior Fitness: Conditioning for Martial Arts

Warrior Fitness will help you and your students attain a new level of strength, flexibility and endurance — quickly and with little chance of injury. **Warrior Fitness combines old school fitness with modern exercise science.**

Guide to Striking Power – **Specific Physical Preparedness for ALL striking arts from old school Traditional Martial Arts to modern MMA!** Learn how to build a powerful structure to stabilize punches, kicks, and martial movement! Discover how to use low-tech, high yield tools to strengthen strikes throughout a range of motion!

Martial Power Program (e-book and video)

The Martial Power Program is for those traditional martial artists committed to taking their body, mind, and spirit to the next level! This program is for people who are serious about learning how to functionally integrate high level fitness training into their martial arts practice!

Ninja Mission Program 1 (Video and Manual)

You will train like the ninja of feudal Japan preparing body, mind, and spirit through rigorous physical training and martial practice

Evolve Your Breathing: Essential Techniques for Optimal Performance

Learn unique and powerful breathing exercises drawn from martial arts, qigong, and yoga that will teach you how to **Adapt AND Perform Under Stress!**

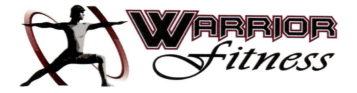

www.WarriorFitness.org

Printed in Great Britain
by Amazon